7 STEPS TO GET OFF SUGAR AND CARBS

ASHLEY CLARK

Copyright page

Copyright © [2023] by [Ashley Clark]

All rights reserved.

TABLE OF CONTENTS

Do you find yourself reaching for sugary or starchy foods all day? Despite getting adequate sleep, do you regularly feel sluggish, weary, or irritable? If so, you might be one of the millions of individuals who are battling with a sugar and carbohydrate-rich diet.

The reality is that sugar and carbs have become so common in our contemporary diet that they are very difficult to avoid. It may be difficult to make healthy food choices, from the sweets we indulge in to the bread and pasta we consume as part of our regular meals.

A high-sugar and high-carbohydrate diet, on the other hand, may have serious repercussions.

It may not only cause weight gain and obesity, but it can also raise the risk of chronic illnesses such as diabetes, heart disease, and even cancer. Furthermore, a high-sugar, high-carbohydrate diet may have a negative impact on your mental health, causing mood swings, anxiety, and sadness.

That is why it is necessary to take action and permanently abstain from sweets and carbs. And the good news is that it is perfectly feasible to do so with a few easy actions and a willingness to change.

This book will teach you the seven fundamental actions you must take to eliminate sugar and carbs from your diet and begin living a better, more energetic life.

From reducing your intake of sugary drinks to increasing your intake of healthy fats and protein, you'll find useful suggestions and guidance to help you make the move to a better lifestyle.

But it's crucial to realize that cutting off sugar and carbs isn't a quick remedy. It is a long-term commitment to making healthy choices and caring for your body and mind.

Following the seven stages suggested in this book will not only improve your general well-being but will also improve your emotional wellness, resulting in a happier, more satisfying existence.

So, if you're ready to take charge of your diet and kick sugar and carbs to the curb, let's get started!

STEP 1

1.1 Avoid Sugary Beverages.

Do you start your day with a cup of sweetened coffee or a can of soda? Or do you grab for an energy drink in the afternoon when you're tired? If this is the case, you are not alone. Sugary drinks have become a mainstay in our contemporary diet, and they are often the source of our sugar cravings and energy dumps during the day.

However, sugary drinks are one of the leading causes of our sugar and carbohydrate overconsumption. They are not only heavy in empty calories, but also high in added sugars, which may be harmful to your health. Sugary drinks may have major effects for your general health, ranging from weight gain to an increased risk of chronic illnesses such as diabetes and heart disease.

That's why the first step in avoiding sugar and carbs is to cut out sugary drinks from your diet. In this chapter, you'll discover why sugary drinks are so bad for your health and practical ways to cut down.

You'll discover easy tactics that will help you break away from your sugary beverage habit for good, such as switching to healthier options and preparing your own flavored water at home.

1.2 The Perils of Sugary Drinks

Soda, sugary coffee and tea, fruit juices, sports drinks, and energetic drinks are all examples of sugary beverages. While they may taste good, they may have major health effects.

They contribute to obesity and weight gain.

One of the most serious risks of sugary beverages is that they contribute to weight gain and obesity. Sugary beverages are high in calories and do not make you feel full or satiated as solid meals do.

As a consequence, it's simple to take a lot of calories from sugary drinks without even recognizing it. People who routinely consume sugary beverages have a greater risk of obesity and an increase in weight than those who do not.

They raise your chances of developing type 2 diabetes.

Sugary beverages have also been related to a higher incidence of type 2 diabetes. When you drink sugary beverages, your body absorbs the sugar quickly, creating an increase in blood sugar levels. This may develop to insulin resistance, a condition whereby your body no longer responds appropriately to insulin. Insulin resistance is a major risk factor for developing type 2 diabetes.

They may cause tooth damage.

Drinking sugary beverages on a frequent basis might potentially harm your teeth. The sugar in these drinks feeds the bacteria in your mouth, causing them to generate acid that destroys your tooth enamel. Cavities, tooth decay, and other dental issues might result from this.

They raise your chances of developing chronic diseases.

Sugary beverages have been associated with an increased risk of chronic illnesses such as heart disease, stroke, and cancer, in addition to the dangers outlined above. This is due to the fact that excessive sugar consumption may promote inflammation in the body, which can contribute to the development of various illnesses.

The risks of sugary beverages cannot be overstated. You may dramatically enhance your health and lower your risk of chronic illnesses by removing sugary drinks from your diet. In the next part, we'll look at some practical suggestions for cutting down on sugary beverages and choosing better choices.

1.3 Sugary Beverage Substitutes

Eliminating sugary beverages from your diet might be difficult, particularly if you're accustomed to drinking them on a daily basis. The good news is that there are several sugar-free options that may help you break the habit and minimize your sugar consumption.

Water

Water is the finest sugar-free substitute for sugary beverages since it is calorie-free, hydrating, and necessary for your body's proper functioning. Water may also help you feel full and minimize your cravings for sugary drinks. According to one research, persons who drank 1-3 glasses of water before meals lost greater significance than those who did not.

If you find water boring, there are several methods to spice it up. Try adding some fresh fruit slices to your glass, such as lemon or cucumber, or investing in a fruit infuser water bottle. You might also try water that bubbles, which is carbonated but has no sugar or calories.

Staying hydrated is critical for your overall health, and the easiest method to do so is to drink water. Make water your preferred beverage, and aim for at least 8 glasses each day. This will not only help you remove sweet beverages from your diet, but it will also improve your digestion, increase your energy, and keep your skin looking healthy.

Teas with Herbs

Herbal teas are another great alternative to sugary beverages. They are available in a variety of tastes, and many are naturally sweet, making them a suitable substitute for sugary drinks. Herbal teas provide several health advantages, including inflammation reduction, digestive help, and relaxation.

Chamomile, peppermint, and ginger are among popular herbal teas. Chamomile tea has relaxing effects and might help you relax before going to bed. Peppermint tea is cooling and might help with digestion. Ginger tea has anti-inflammatory properties and may help reduce nausea.

Simply steep the tea bag or loose leaves in boiling water for 3-5 minutes to produce herbal teas. Depending on your inclination, you can eat them hot or cold. If you find them too bitter, try a dash of honey or a squeeze of lemon to give some natural sweetness.

Coffee and tea without sugar

If you consume coffee or tea, switch to unsweetened kinds. If desired, add a splash of milk or cream, but leave off the sugar and flavored syrups. This will drastically cut your sugar consumption and assist you in breaking the habit of drinking sweetened coffee or tea.

When drunk in moderation, coffee and tea provide several health advantages. They are high in antioxidants, which may decrease inflammation, reduce the risk of chronic illnesses, and boost brain function. However, don't overdo it, since too much caffeine might cause jitters and affect your sleep.

Simply boil your preferred mix and add milk or cream if desired to create unsweetened coffee or tea. You may also try various tastes like chai or green tea. Just keep in mind to avoid using sugar or artificial sweeteners.

Sparkling Water with Flavors

If you want the carbonation of soda, try flavored sparkling water. Many businesses provide unsweetened versions flavored with natural fruit extracts. This gives you the zing you want without the extra sugar and calories of soda.

Flavored sparkling water is an excellent method to alleviate thirst and fulfill appetites without ingesting too much sugar. It's also a healthy substitute for regular soda, which has been attributed to weight gain, diabetes, and other health problems.

Simply pour flavored sparkling water into a cup with ice and enjoy. You may also add a slice of lemon or lime for a taste boost.

Alternatives to Milk

If you like milk-based beverages like lattes or hot chocolate, consider milk substitutes like almond milk, soy milk, or oat milk. These dairy-free alternatives have less sugar and calories than regular milk and may be used in a number of recipes. They're also high in vitamins and minerals like calcium and vitamin D, both of which are essential for bone health.

When selecting a milk substitute, check the labels carefully and avoid those with additional sugars.

Look for unsweetened types that are nutrient-fortified. Almond milk is a popular choice since it has few calories and has a nutty taste that complements coffee and tea.

Soy milk is another fantastic option since it is strong in protein and can be used in a variety of dishes. Oat milk is another popular choice since it is creamy and somewhat sweet.

Simply boil the milk in a pot and add the cocoa powder or coffee to produce a latte or hot chocolate with milk alternatives. Milk substitutes may also be used in smoothies, oatmeal, and baking dishes.

Juice that has been freshly squeezed
Make freshly squeezed juice from fruits and vegetables if you're seeking something sweet. This gives natural sweetness as well as important vitamins and minerals. However, keep in mind that fruit juice might still contain a lot of sugar.

When producing juice, aim to use largely vegetables and just a little bit of fruit. This will assist to minimize sugar content while increasing nutritious density. Kale, spinach, cucumber, and celery are all wonderful vegetable choices. Oranges, grapefruit, and berries are other excellent alternatives.

Simply combine the ingredients in a shredder or blender and strain the liquid through a cheesecloth to produce freshly squeezed juice. You may also try other taste combos and combinations to discover your favorite.

You may lower your sugar consumption, keep hydrated, and enhance your overall health by substituting sugary beverages with these healthier options. Try introducing these beverages into your everyday regimen and see how you feel. Remember that tiny adjustments may have a significant impact over time.

Step 2

2.1 Limit your intake of processed foods.

Congratulations for taking the first step toward a better living by avoiding sugary drinks. It's now time to move on to the next step: reducing your intake of processed meals. Processed foods are common in today's diet, however they are typically high in added sugars, salt, and bad fats. You may enhance your general health and lower your risk of chronic illnesses by limiting your intake of processed foods.

In this stage, we'll look at the hazards of processed foods, how to spot them in your diet, and practical ways to cut down on them. Cutting down on processed foods is an important step in attaining your health objectives, whether you want to reduce weight, increase your energy, or just feel better in your body. Let's get started and discover more about how processed foods affect your health.

2.2 What Effects Processed Foods Have on Your Health

Foods that are processed have become an indispensable element of the contemporary diet, yet they are not as harmless as they seem. These meals are often heavy in calories, added sugars, bad fats, and salt, all of which may lead to negative health results. In this part, we'll look at how processed foods affect your health and well-being.

Chronic Disease Risk Increase

One of the most serious risks of processed foods is its link to chronic illnesses including diabetes, heart disease, and cancer. These meals are often heavy in calories, added sugars, and harmful fats, which may lead to weight gain and obesity. Obesity, in turn, is a significant risk factor for chronic illnesses such as type 2 diabetes and cardiovascular disease. Furthermore, many processed meals have high salt levels, which may contribute to high blood pressure and an increased risk of heart disease.

Deficiencies in Nutrients

Another way processed meals might harm your health is by causing vitamin shortages. During the production process, processed foods are often stripped of their natural nutrients and supplemented with synthetic vitamins and minerals.

While these additional nutrients might be useful, they do not provide the same benefits as the natural nutrients found in entire meals. Furthermore, many processed meals are heavy in calories but deficient in vital nutrients like fiber, leaving you feeling hungry and dissatisfied.

Understanding the influence of processed foods on your health allows you to make better educated eating choices. In the next part, we'll look at how to detect processed foods in your diet and give you practical advice on how to cut down on them.

Digestive Issues and Inflammation

Processed meals may also lead to inflammation in the body, which has been linked to a variety of health issues such as arthritis, heart disease, and cancer. Many processed meals include high quantities of refined carbohydrates, which may induce blood sugar spikes and increase inflammation in the body.

Furthermore, many processed meals include artificial preservatives, tastes, and colors that may irritate the digestive system and lead to digestive problems including bloating, gas, and constipation.

Cravings and Addiction

Because of their high sugar, fat, and salt content, processed foods may be very addictive. These meals may cause the brain to produce dopamine, a chemical linked with emotions of pleasure and reward. This may lead to a dependency on processed meals and desires for sweet, fatty, and salty snacks over time. Breaking the cycle of processed food addiction might be difficult, but it is necessary in enhancing your health and wellness.

Knowing how processed foods may harm your health allows you to start making changes to replace them with more healthy whole foods. In the next part, we'll show you how to recognize processed foods in your diet and make better choices.

2.3 Tips for Cutting Back on Processed Foods

Now that we've discussed the hazards of processed meals, let's look at some practical ways to cut down on these unhealthy items. You may enhance your health and wellbeing while lowering your risk of chronic illnesses by adopting a few easy dietary modifications. Here are some suggestions for reducing your intake of processed foods:

Examine Food Labels

Reading product labels is an important step in determining the presence of processed foods in your diet. Choose foods with little processing and entire components, such as fruits and vegetables, whole grains, and lean meats. Foods with added sugars, artificial colors, tastes, and preservatives should be avoided. The components are given in decreasing order of weight, with the first few being the most vital. Choose meals with fewer ingredients and ones that you are familiar with.

Cooking at Home More

Another excellent strategy to limit your consumption of processed foods is to cook more meals at home. You have control over the items you use when you make your meals, and you may pick whole foods that are healthful and fulfilling. Experiment with different recipes and cooking methods, and make an effort to include more fruits, vegetables, healthy grains, and lean meats in your diet. Cooking at home may be a creative and exciting method to enhance your health and well-being.

Whole Foods Snacks

Many of us eat processed snacks all through the day, but they are generally heavy in calories, added sugars, and bad fats. Instead of grabbing for a bag of chips or a candy bar, choose healthy foods like fruits, vegetables, nuts, and seeds. These meals are healthy and filling, and they may keep you energetic and full throughout the day. Keep nutritious snacks on hand so you aren't tempted to grab processed foods when you're hungry.

By following these guidelines, you may begin to minimize your consumption of processed foods while also improving your general health and well-being. Remember that even tiny adjustments to your diet may have a major influence on your health, so start with one or two changes at a time and work your way up.

Shop the Grocery Store's Periphery

Another way to cut less on processed meals is to browse around the perimeter of the market. Whole foods including fruits, vegetables, whole grains, and lean meats may be found here. The center aisles of the grocery store are usually where you'll find processed goods, so try to avoid them as much as possible. Sticking within the store's perimeter allows you to pick more healthful whole foods while avoiding the temptations of packaged snacks and sweets.

When dining out, choose whole foods.

When it comes to avoiding packaged food, eating out might be difficult, but there are still methods to make better choices. Look for places that provide whole meals like salads, grilled veggies, and lean meats.

Dishes that are fried or laden with cheese and creamy sauces should be avoided. Instead of sugary drinks, go for water or unsweetened liquids. You may also request that your waitress make changes to your dish, such as swapping a side salad for fries.

Meal Planning and Preparation

Meal planning and preparation might help you limit your consumption of processed foods. You'll be less inclined to depend on processed foods when you prepare meals ahead of time. Schedule your meals for the week and create a shopping list of nutritious foods.

Set aside time each week to plan ahead of time for meals and snacks, such as cutting vegetables, cooking grains, and preparing salads. This will assist you in staying on track and making better choices all through the week.

You may enhance your health and wellbeing while lowering your risk of chronic illnesses by following these guidelines for eliminating processed foods. Remember that progress, not perfection, is the goal. Begin with simple dietary adjustments and work your way up. You may adopt healthy eating habits and get the advantages of a nutritious diet with time and persistence.

Step 3

3.1 Increase Your Protein Consumption

Increasing your protein consumption is an excellent place to start if you want to enhance your health and nutrition. Protein is a food that is important for numerous biological activities, including tissue growth and repair, immune function support, and hormone regulation.

Furthermore, protein may help you feel satisfied for longer, which can assist with weight reduction and control. In this stage, we'll look at the advantages of protein and give you some recommendations for increasing your protein consumption in a way that is environmentally friendly and sustainable.

Increasing your protein consumption may have several advantages, whether you're an athlete wanting to gain muscle or just looking to enhance your general health. Protein is an essential component of any healthy diet, since it aids in muscle development and repair, boosts metabolism, and makes you feel full. So, let's get started and learn more about increasing your protein consumption to boost your health and wellness.

3.2 Why Is Protein Important?

Protein is an important food that is required for numerous body activities. It is, in fact, one of the three macronutrients that our systems need in big quantities, along with carbs and fats. Here are a few of the reasons why protein is so beneficial to your health:

Tissue Formation and Repair

Protein is required for the formation and repair of tissues throughout the body, including muscles, bones, skin, and hair. When you eat protein, it has been divided into amino acids, which are the protein's building components. These amino acids are used by your body to make new tissues and repair damaged ones. Protein is especially essential for athletes and those who participate in regular physical exercise because their bodies need extra protein to maintain muscle development and repair.

Immune Function Support

Protein is also necessary for immunological function. Proteins are the building blocks of many immune cells, including antibodies and cytokines. These proteins aid in the identification and destruction of microorganisms that cause infections and diseases, such as viruses and bacteria. Furthermore, protein is essential for wound healing since it aids in the formation of new tissues and the repair of damaged ones.

Hormone Administration

Protein is essential for hormone regulation in your body. Hormones are substances generated by glands and organs throughout the body. They aid in the regulation of various biological activities, such as metabolism, growth and development, and reproduction. Many hormones, including insulin and growth hormone, are composed of proteins. Your body may be unable to manufacture or regulate these hormones adequately if you do not consume enough protein.

Helping with Weight Loss

Protein may also help you lose weight. Protein, unlike carbs and fats, takes longer to digest, so it might help you feel full for extended periods of time. This might help you cut your total calorie consumption and make sticking to a healthy eating plan simpler. Furthermore, protein has a larger thermic impact than carbs and lipids, which means your body expends more calories digesting and processing protein than other foods.

Brain Function Support

Protein is required for brain function. To operate effectively, your brain requires a regular supply of glucose, which is produced by the breakdown of carbs. Protein, on the other hand, is necessary for the formation of neurotransmitters, which are substances that convey impulses in your brain. Dopamine, for example, is derived from the amino acid tyrosine, which is abundant in protein-rich diets.

Blood Pressure Reduction

Increasing your protein intake may also aid in blood pressure reduction. Protein-rich diets, especially plant-based proteins like beans and lentils, have been demonstrated in studies to help lower blood pressure. This is due to the fact that protein has been demonstrated to increase the function of the endothelium, the inner lining of blood vessels. Improving endothelial function may aid in increased blood flow and blood pressure reduction.

3.3 How to Get More Protein into Your Diet

There are several strategies to integrate additional protein into your diet, whether you consume meat or are a vegetarian or vegan. Here are some pointers to help you increase your protein intake:

Select Protein-Rich Foods

Choosing protein-rich meals is the easiest approach to improve your protein consumption. Some of the most popular protein sources include animal-based proteins such as meat, poultry, fish, and eggs. If you're a vegetarian or vegan, there are lots of plant-based protein sources to choose from, such as beans, lentils, nuts, and seeds. Protein-rich dairy products, such as Greek yogurt and cottage cheese, are additional options.

Protein First Thing in the Morning
Starting your day with a high-protein breakfast will help you feel full and energetic throughout the day. Eggs, Greek yogurt, and protein smoothies prepared with protein powder, fruit, and milk or yogurt are other protein-rich breakfast alternatives. If you don't have time, grab a protein bar or prepare overnight oats with Greek yogurt and nuts or seeds.

Protein should be packed for snacks.
Many snack foods are strong in carbs and low in protein, leaving you hungry shortly after eating. To overcome this, carry protein-rich snacks between meals to keep you feeling full. Hard-boiled eggs,

beef jerky, string cheese, and hummus with vegetables or crackers are also healthy alternatives.

Include Protein in Your Meals

You may also include protein-rich items into your dishes to boost protein to your meals. Beans and lentils, for example, may be added to soups and stews, salads can be topped with grilled chicken or fish, and stir-fries can be made with tofu or tempeh. Protein-rich snacks and sweets may also be produced, such as protein balls made with nuts and protein powder or Greek yogurt with fruit and honey.

You may improve your health and feel more satiated after meals by including extra protein in your diet. With these techniques, you may quickly boost your protein consumption and get the many advantages it provides.

Step 4

4.1 Consume More Healthy Fats

If you want to enhance your health and nutrition, one crucial step is to include a greater amount of benefits in your meals. While many people equate fat with weight gain and bad health, the fact is that certain fats are really beneficial to your health and required for normal biological function. This phase will teach you why healthy fats are necessary and how to include them in your diet.

Eating more healthy fats may provide a variety of health advantages. It may help you feel more pleased and full after meals, as well as boost cognitive function, decrease inflammation, and lessen your risk of chronic illnesses including heart disease and diabetes. You can experience these advantages and promote your general health and well-being by recognizing the various kinds of fats and making a few easy modifications to your diet.

4.2 Heart Health Advantages of Healthy Fats

Fats that are healthy such as those found in avocados, nuts and seeds, and fatty seafood, may help improve heart health. Monounsaturated and polyunsaturated fats have been demonstrated in studies to decrease LDL cholesterol levels, improve blood pressure, and lessen the risk of heart disease.

Furthermore, omega-3 fatty acids, which are abundant in fatty fish, have been related to decreased triglyceride levels and a lower incidence of arrhythmias.

Healthy fats are necessary for optimum brain function and growth. The brain is mainly fat, and omega-3 fatty acids are especially crucial for cognitive function and lowering the risk of neurodegenerative disorders such as Alzheimer's and dementia. Increasing omega-3 consumption has been demonstrated in studies to enhance memory, mood, and attention.

Weight Management

Contrary to common perception, eating healthy fats may help you lose weight. Healthy fats improve satiety, which means you will feel fuller for longer and will be less prone to overeat. They may also help manage blood sugar levels and lower insulin resistance, both of which can contribute to weight growth.

Chronic inflammation has been related to a variety of health issues such as heart disease, diabetes, and arthritis. Consuming healthy fats, on the other hand, may help decrease inflammation in the body. Omega-3 fatty acids, in particular, have been demonstrated to have anti-inflammatory properties and may aid in the treatment of illnesses such as rheumatoid arthritis and inflammatory bowel disease.

Adding healthy fats into your diet may offer a variety of health and well-being advantages. These essential elements should be a regular component of your diet for a variety of reasons, including improved heart health and cognitive function, weight control, and inflammation reduction.

4.3 Healthy Fats to Include in Your Diet Examples

When it comes to introducing more beneficial fats into your diet, it's critical to understand which kinds of fats to prioritize. Here are some examples of healthy fats to incorporate in your diet:

Avocados are high in heart-healthy monounsaturated fats, which have been linked to decreased cholesterol levels and better heart health. These healthy fats also enhance satiety, so you'll be full and pleased after consuming them. Avocados also include a lot of fiber, potassium, and vitamins C and K. Avocados may be readily included into your diet by adding slices to salads, sandwiches, or toast. Guacamole may also be used as a dip for vegetables or tortilla chips, or blended into smoothies for a creamy texture.

Nuts and seeds are high in good fats, protein, fiber, and other critical components. They've been proved to help with heart health, inflammation, and even weight reduction.

Almonds, for example, have a high concentration of monounsaturated fats and vitamin E, while chia seeds have a high concentration of omega-3 fatty acids, fiber, and antioxidants. To add extra nuts and seeds to your diet, sprinkle them on top of cereal or yogurt, or add them to smoothies for a crunchy texture. You can also eat them on their own as a snack or prepare your own nut butter to put over toast or use as a dip.

Fatty fish, such as salmon, mackerel, and tuna, are high in omega-3 fatty acids, which are necessary for brain function, heart health, and inflammation reduction. These good fats have been found to boost mood, mental abilities, and even lower the risk of some chronic illnesses.

Aim to consume fatty fish at least twice a week to increase your intake. You may bake or broil them and serve them with roasted veggies or a salad on the side. If you don't like fish, consider taking supplements containing omega-3 fatty acids to receive the advantages of these vital fats.

STEP 5

5.1 Select Complex Carbohydrates

One of the finest things you can do to enhance your diet and general health is to pick complex carbs over simple carbohydrates. While simple carbohydrates provide a brief surge of energy, they may also cause blood sugar rises and leave you feeling hungry shortly afterwards. Complex carbohydrates, on the other hand, give long-lasting energy as well as a number of essential elements. Step 5 will go over the advantages of complex carbohydrates and how to include them into your diet.

You may boost your energy levels, lower your risk of chronic illnesses, and maintain a healthy weight by switching to complex carbs. However, with so many various kinds of carbohydrates available, it might be difficult to know which ones to select. That's why we'll go over the distinctions between complex and simple carbohydrates, as well as some simple and tasty methods to integrate complex carbs into your everyday meals. So, prepare to feel your best by eating complex carbs.

5.2 What Exactly Are Complex Carbohydrates?

Carbohydrates, along with protein and fat, are one of the three macronutrients that make up the food we consume. Complex carbohydrates are composed of lengthy chains of sugar molecules that take longer to break down and release energy at a slower pace than simple carbs. These chains are composed of three kinds of carbohydrates: starch, fiber, and glycogen.

Complex Carbohydrate Types

The most prevalent form of complex carb is starch, which may be found in whole grains, legumes, and starchy vegetables like potatoes and maize.

These meals also include fiber, which is an indigestible component of plant foods that helps you feel full and promotes good digestion. Glycogen, on the other hand, is a complex carbohydrate that is stored as an energy source in your muscles and liver.

Eating a complex carbohydrate-rich diet may bring several health advantages, including improved digestion, increased cognitive function, and a decreased risk of chronic illnesses.

A diet heavy in simple carbs, such as those found in processed foods and sugary beverages, on the other hand, may result in weight gain, insulin resistance, and an increased risk of heart disease and type 2 diabetes.

Complex Carbohydrate Examples

Whole grains like brown rice, quinoa, and oatmeal, as well as fruits, vegetables, and legumes like lentils and chickpeas, are rich in complex carbs. These meals not only include nutrients such as fiber, vitamins, and minerals, but they also give a continuous supply of energy throughout the day.

5.3 How to Add Complex Carbohydrates to Your Diet

Now that you know how important complex carbs are, it's time to figure out how to include them into your diet. Here are some pointers to get you started:

Select Whole Grain Foods

When shopping for bread, pasta, cereal, and other grain-based meals, search for whole grain selections. Because the grain has not been processed, it has all three components: bran, germ, and endosperm. Whole grain meals are high in fiber, vitamins, and minerals, and they may help you feel satisfied for extended periods of time.

Increase your intake of vegetables and fruits.

Vegetables and fruits are high in complex carbs, fiber, vitamins, and minerals. Include a range of colorful fruits and vegetables in your daily meals and snacks. Try incorporating veggies into your omelets, salads, or soups, or munch on fresh fruit between meals.

Don't Forget About Legumes

Legumes, such as lentils, chickpeas, and black beans, are high in complex carbs, protein, and fiber. Make vegetarian chili, add them to salads, or use them as a meat alternative in tacos or burritos to include more beans into your meals.

Keep Portion Sizes in Mind

While complex carbohydrates are an essential element of a balanced diet, portion proportions must be considered. Eating too many carbs of any kind may lead to an increase in weight and other health issues. Half of your plate should include vegetables and fruits, a quarter complete grains or legumes, and a quarter protein-rich meals.

You may simply integrate more complex carbs into your diet and get numerous health advantages by following these guidelines.

STEP 6

6.1 Exercise on a regular basis.

Regular exercise is essential for a healthy lifestyle, and it may be a powerful tool for weaning yourself off sweets and carbs. Exercise burns calories, reduces stress, and increases metabolism, all of which may help you reach your weight reduction objectives.

Exercise has been demonstrated to boost mental health, lower the risk of chronic illnesses, and increase general wellbeing, in addition to its physical advantages.

If you're trying to cut down on sugar and carbs, including regular exercise into your routine may be a great aid in helping you attain your objectives.

However, knowing where to begin and how to maintain a regular workout regimen may be difficult. In this part, we'll go over the advantages of regular exercise, different forms of exercise to think about, and ways to keep motivated. We've got you covered whether you're new to fitness or trying to get back into a regimen.

6.2 How Exercise Aids in the Treatment of Sugar and Carbohydrate Cravings

One of the most effective strategies to enhance your general health and well-being is to exercise. It has a plethora of advantages, including weight reduction, better cardiovascular health, enhanced energy levels, and less stress and anxiety.

One of the lesser-known advantages of exercise is that it may help lower sugar and carbohydrate cravings. In this part, we'll look at how exercise may help you conquer sugar and carb cravings, as well as give you some pointers on how to include exercise into your daily routine.

Endorphins are released during exercise, which reduces cravings.

Endorphins are released during exercise, which is one of the reasons why it may help reduce sugar and carbohydrate cravings.

Endorphins are the body's natural "feel-good" chemicals that may assist to relieve stress and anxiety, both of which can contribute to cravings. Exercise causes your body to release more endorphins, which may aid in the reduction of cravings for sweets and other harmful foods.

Endorphins, in addition to lowering cravings, may improve your mood and energy levels, making it simpler to adhere to your healthy eating plan. Exercise may help to decrease stress and anxiety, improve your mood and energy levels, and lessen cravings for sugary and carb-heavy meals.

Insulin sensitivity is improved by exercise.

Exercise may also assist to lower sugar and carb cravings by enhancing insulin sensitivity. When you consume sugary or carb-heavy meals, your body produces insulin to assist move the sugar from your circulation into your cells.

However, eating too many sugary or carb-heavy meals might cause your body to grow resistant to insulin, resulting in a condition known as insulin resistance. Insulin resistance is linked to a variety of chronic diseases, including type 2 diabetes, heart disease, and obesity.

Regular exercise may help to increase insulin sensitivity, lowering your risk of insulin resistance and the health issues that come with it. Exercise may help manage blood sugar levels by boosting insulin sensitivity, lowering cravings for sugar and other harmful meals.

Exercise improves restful sleep.
Finally, exercise may aid in the promotion of sound sleep, which can be beneficial in minimizing sugar and carb cravings. When you don't get enough sleep, your body creates more ghrelin, a hormone that increases hunger and may lead to desires for unhealthy foods.

Exercise has been demonstrated to increase sleep quality and duration, which may aid in the reduction of ghrelin levels and cravings for sugary and carb-heavy diets. You may help to minimize cravings and enhance your general health and well-being by obtaining regular exercise and optimizing your sleeping patterns.

6.3 How to Begin an Exercise Routine

Begin slowly and gradually increase your intensity.

One of the most common errors individuals make when beginning an exercise plan is attempting to do too much too soon. Starting softly and progressively increasing the intensity of your exercises over time is critical. Not only does this assist avoid injury, but it also enables your body to adapt and get stronger.

Begin your workout program with low-impact activities such as walking, swimming, or yoga. Begin with a short period and modest intensity, gradually increasing both as you gain comfort. A decent rule of thumb is to only increase your exercise duration or intensity by 10% every week.

Find an Exercise That You Like.

Finding an activity that you like is one of the keys to adhering to a workout plan. Because there are so many various sorts of exercise to select from, it's important to explore and discover what works best for you. Some individuals like jogging, while others enjoy weightlifting or dancing.

If you don't know where to begin, try a few different things to discover what you like. It's also crucial to switch things up and diversify your exercises to avoid boredom and to push your body in new ways.

You may discover that you love group exercise courses, outdoor activities such as hiking or cycling, or home workouts using internet videos or apps. The idea is to discover something you like doing and that works into your schedule.

Set attainable objectives.

Setting realistic objectives is critical for remaining motivated and progressing in your fitness regimen. It's important to have a clear vision of what you want to accomplish, but it's also critical to be practical and create objectives that are attainable.

Consider what you want to achieve in the short and long term while developing objectives. Short-term objectives may include increasing your training duration or frequency, whilst long-term goals could involve running a 5K or lifting a specific amount of weight. Make your objectives concrete, quantifiable, and time-bound, and divide them into smaller segments that you can work on each week.

Make it a habit to exercise.

To get the advantages of exercise, it is necessary to make it a habit. This involves making your exercises a non-negotiable part of your routine and scheduling them at the same time every day or week. It also entails finding methods to include exercise into your regular routine, such as walking or cycling to work instead of driving.

Making exercise a habit requires making a strategy and sticking to it.
Make a weekly fitness routine and block off time in your calendar so that nothing else interferes.

Finding an accountability partner or joining a fitness group may also be beneficial in keeping you motivated and on track. Remember that the more you practice exercise, the simpler it will become with time.

STEP 7

7.1 Get Enough Sleep

Getting adequate sleep is an important element of living a healthy lifestyle, yet it is sometimes disregarded. Many individuals put their job and social activities above their sleep, which leads to the harmful consequences of sleep deprivation. In this last part of our sugar and carb detox program, we will discuss the significance of sleep and how it may help you reach your health objectives.

Adequate sleep is essential for physical and mental health because it helps your body to relax, recover, and repair itself. Sleep deprivation may result in a number of poor health effects, including weight gain, lowered immunity, and diminished cognitive performance.

Furthermore, sleep deprivation increases your chances of acquiring chronic health issues including diabetes and heart disease. You may enhance your general health and well-being by prioritizing your sleep, making it simpler to follow the other recommendations in this program.

7.2 Sleep and Sugar Cravings: A Connection

Sleep quality and length may influence food desires and appetite, especially when it comes to sweet meals. Sleep deprivation may affect appetite-controlling hormones, leading to an increased craving for high-calorie, high-sugar meals. Step 7 will investigate the relationship between sleep and sugar cravings and teach you how to enhance your sleep to lessen sugar cravings.

Sleep and Hormones

Sleep deprivation may have an impact on the hormones that control your appetite. Sleep deprivation causes an increase in the hormone ghrelin, which promotes appetite, and a reduction in the hormone leptin, which communicates feelings of fullness. This hormonal imbalance may cause an increase in hunger as well as a desire for high-calorie, high-sugar meals.

Furthermore, sleep is essential for blood sugar management. Sleep deprivation may impair the body's capacity to control blood sugar, resulting in increased glucose levels in the circulation. This may lead to insulin resistance, a disease in which the body becomes less sensitive to insulin and is unable to adequately manage blood sugar. Insulin resistance has been linked to an increased risk of type 2 diabetes, obesity, and metabolic syndrome.

The Importance of Good Sleep

Getting enough sleep is crucial, but so is the quality of sleep. Deep sleep, sometimes referred to as slow-wave sleep, is necessary for the body's restoration and repair processes. The body releases growth hormone during this period of sleep, which is required for tissue repair and muscular development.

Poor-quality sleep, on the other hand, such as interrupted sleep or a lack of deep sleep, may contribute to a variety of health issues, including an increased risk of chronic illnesses such as obesity, diabetes, and heart disease.

Furthermore, lack of sleep may raise stress levels, resulting in an increased craving for high-sugar, high-calorie meals.

Improving the quality and length of your sleep may help you lose weight and improve your overall health. In the next part, we'll look at some recommendations and tactics for improving the quality and length of your sleep.

7.3 Methods for Getting More Sleep

Maintain a Regular Sleep Schedule

Consistency is as vital as getting adequate sleep each night. Your body can create a regular sleep cycle if you go to bed and get up at the same time every day.

This may aid in the regulation of your hormones, especially those that govern hunger and appetite. Maintaining a consistent sleep pattern may reduce your chances of experiencing sugar cravings caused by hormonal imbalances produced by inconsistent sleep.

Try to go to bed and get up at the same time every day, including on weekends, to maintain a regular sleep routine. You may set an alarm to remind you when it's time to sleep and when it's time to get up.

On weekends, avoid staying up too late or sleeping in too much, since this may disturb your sleep routine and make it difficult to keep to throughout the week. Sticking to a steady sleep pattern may help lower sugar cravings and enhance your overall health over time.

Make a Calming Bedtime Routine

Stress and worry may make it harder to fall and remain asleep, affecting your general health and increasing your chances of developing sugar cravings.

You may help quiet your thoughts and prepare your body for sleep by developing a soothing nighttime ritual. Activities like having a warm bath, reading a book, or practicing relaxation methods such as deep breathing or meditation may all contribute to this.

Establish a consistent bedtime ritual that you follow each night before bed to build a soothing evening habit. This might tell your body that it's time to relax and prepare for sleep. You should also avoid devices and bright lights before going to bed since they might disrupt the synthesis of melatonin, a hormone that helps regulate sleep. Instead, use dark illumination or relaxation methods to relax. A soothing nighttime practice may help enhance the quality of your sleep and lower your risk of sugar cravings over time.

Establish a regular sleeping schedule.

This includes going to bed and getting up at the same time every day, including weekends. Our bodies thrive on consistency, and sticking to a sleep plan may help regulate your circadian cycle, making it easier to sleep and get up naturally.

Developing a soothing nighttime ritual may also aid in the preparation of your mind and body for sleep. Taking a warm bath or shower, reading a book, doing moderate yoga or stretching, or listening to peaceful music are all examples.

Avoiding stimulating activities such as utilizing technology or indulging in stressful work-related chores before bed might keep your mind attentive and make it difficult to fall asleep.

Creating a peaceful evening ritual and establishing a sleep habit

It is critical to establish a sleep-friendly atmosphere. Make your bedroom as dark, quiet, and chilly as possible. To create a pleasant sleeping environment, consider utilizing blackout curtains, earplugs, a white noise machine, or a fan.

You should also consider purchasing a comfy mattress and pillows to support your body and keep you comfortable during the night. You may enhance your sleep quality and lower your risk of sugar cravings induced by sleep loss by prioritizing sleep and establishing a pleasant sleep environment.

Conclusion

As we near the conclusion of this book, it is crucial to highlight the importance of the seven stages given to assist you in breaking your sugar and carbohydrate addiction. With the abundance of sugar and carbohydrate-filled items in our diets, breaking the addiction cycle may be difficult. You may, however, make the required adjustments to lead a healthy lifestyle with determination and commitment.

To summarize, the seven phases stated in this book are as follows: Understand how sugar and carbs affect your body. Reduce your consumption of processed foods. Increase your protein consumption.

Consume more healthful fats and complex carbs. Get adequate sleep and exercise on a regular basis. Each of these stages is important in assisting you to conquer your sugar and carbohydrate cravings. You may make better choices, increase your energy, and reach your health objectives by following these steps.

It is important to remember that living a sugar and carbohydrate-free diet is a continuous effort that demands dedication and persistence. While it may be difficult at first, your body will adapt to these adjustments and you will begin to experience the advantages. Remember to be patient with yourself and to acknowledge your accomplishments along the road.

Finally, the seven stages indicated in this book provide a realistic roadmap to overcoming sugar and carbohydrate addiction. You may enhance your general health and well-being and live a more happy life by following these tips. Remember, the route to a better lifestyle starts with the first step, and you can reach your health objectives with commitment, determination, and the appropriate mentality.